43 Meal Recipes to Improve Your Eye Sight:

Feed Your Body Vitamin Rich Foods That Will Help You Strengthen Your Eye Sight and Prevent Loss of Vision

By

Joe Correa CSN

COPYRIGHT

ACKNOWLEDGEMENTS

This book is dedicated to my friends and family that have had mild or serious illnesses so that you may find a solution and make the necessary changes in your life.

43 Meal Recipes to Improve Your Eye Sight:

Feed Your Body Vitamin Rich Foods That Will Help You Strengthen Your Eye Sight and Prevent Loss of Vision

By

Joe Correa CSN

CONTENTS

ABOUT THE AUTHOR

After years of Research, I honestly believe in the positive effects that proper nutrition can have over the body and mind. My knowledge and experience has helped me live healthier throughout the years and which I have shared with family and friends. The more you know about eating and drinking healthier, the sooner you will want to change your life and eating habits.

Nutrition is a key part in the process of being healthy and living longer so get started today. The first step is the most important and the most significant.

INTRODUCTION

43 Meal Recipes to Improve Your Eye Sight: Feed Your Body Vitamin Rich Foods That Will Help You Strengthen Your Eye Sight and Prevent Loss of Vision

By Joe Correa CSN

Have you ever caught yourself in a market or on the street where you simply can't read the product label or a street sign? Sooner or later, this happens to all of us. Losing eye sight is a normal process of aging and most people don't pay much attention to it. Just a few generations ago, wearing eyeglasses was reserved only for older people, but times are changing. More and more young people are losing their eye sight. A modern lifestyle that requires the use of cell phones and computers, combined with a lack of exercise and proper nutrition makes it hard to maintain healthy eyes. This doesn't mean that you should accept seeing blurry every time you want to read something. Doing more exercise outdoors and eating better can greatly improve your vision and prevent future loss of eye sight. This book will help you to take care of the nutrition portion of protecting your eyes since it will give you some of the best eye sight specific recipes you can find.

We can't deny the fact that our work is mostly in front of computers. This goes on and on every day for at least 8 hours, but we can do our best to help our body heal through nutrition. Eye sight is a precious gift without any known replacement which is exactly why you should take this problem seriously.

The first thing you should do for yourself is to avoid any unnecessary time in front of the tv, computer, and other devices. These things are proven to be harmful for your eyes and is also the number one reason for losing eye sight. Instead of spending the afternoon watching tv, consider taking a walk with your dog or going out for a run.

Some simple changes in your diet can have significant changes in your health. Hippocrates once said: "Let food be thy medicine and medicine be thy food." This is so true! A proper diet is definitely a mucheasier way to prevent eye problems and so many other different dieseases and conditions. Its influence on eye sight is often unjustly neglected because most people blame these problems with too much time on the computer or cell phone. This is true, but just like everything else, there is a lot you can do from the inside to help your body heal and strengthen on the outside. A lack of nutrients in early childhood has proven to cause eye sight problems in adulthood. This means that there is a lot you can do to help yourself and your family to prevent this problem early on.

This cookbook contains delicious recipes prepared with precisely chosen ingredients that will help keep your eye sight health in check. Vegetables like carrots, spinach, kale, and other leafy greens are natural antioxidants that will boost your eye nutrition and overall health.

Legumes, on the other hand, are full of precious zinc, while beans are a perfect source of bioflavonoids that prevent and lower the risk of eye health complications.

Omega-3 fatty acids can be found in fish like salmon, mackerel, and tuna. Omegas are really one of the best medicines you can possibly find in food, but when you combine them with a huge amount of vitamin A in Salmon with Carrots, you create a great combination of nutrients for your eyes.

All orange, red, and yellow vegetables are really a great source of carotenoids which is one of the best-known compounds for eye health. This is exactly why I have collected plenty of recipes based on tomatoes, sweet potatoes, carrots, and bell peppers. These recipes are healthy and tasty but at the same time will do a great job to protect your eyes.

I truly hope you will find this book useful for your entire family. Eye sight is a precious gift from nature so don't waste it!

43 MEAL RECIPES TO IMPROVE YOUR EYE SIGHT: FEED YOUR BODY VITAMIN RICH FOODS THAT WILL HELP YOU STRENGTHEN YOUR EYE SIGHT AND PREVENT LOSS OF VISION

1. Salmon with Carrots

Ingredients:

1 lb of salmon filets, skinless and boneless

4 large carrots, sliced

1 cup of spinach, chopped

2 tbsp of lemon juice

3 tbsp of olive oil

3 garlic cloves, chopped

½ tsp of salt

¼ tsp of black pepper, ground

1 tbsp of balsamic vinegar

1 tbsp of fresh rosemary, finely chopped

Preparation:

Preheat the oven to 375°F.

Combine vinegar, 2 tablespoons of oil, lemon juice,rosemary, salt, and pepper in a large glass bowl. Add meat and coat well. Refrigerate for 15 minutes to allow flavors to penetrate into the meat.

Place some baking paper on a large baking sheet. Spread the carrot slices and garlic onto the bottom and top with meat. Put it in the oven and bake for 15 minutes, or until doneness. Remove from the oven and serve with lemon wedges or extra rosemary to taste.

Nutrition information per serving: Kcal: 280, Protein: 23.1g, Carbs: 8.9g, Fats: 17.7g

2. Orange Salad

Ingredients:

4 large oranges, chopped

2 cups of Romaine lettuce, chopped

¼ cup of raisins

2 medium-sized apple, cored and chopped

1 medium-sized carrot, sliced

1 cup of Greek yogurt

1 tbsp of lemon juice

½ tsp of salt

¼ tsp of Cayenne pepper, ground

Preparation:

Combine yogurt,lemon juice, salt, and pepper in a mixing bowl. Stir to combine and set aside.

Combine oranges, lettuce, apple, carrot, and raisins in a salad bowl. Toss well and drizzle with marinade. Give it a good stir and refrigerate for 30 minutes. Sprinkle with fresh mint before serving.

Nutrition information per serving: Kcal: 147, Protein: 5.1g, Carbs: 32.4g, Fats: 1.0g

3. Green Pasta

Ingredients:

1 lb of broccoli, chopped

1 lb of pasta, pre-cooked

½ cup of lemon juice, freshly squeezed

2 tbsp of fresh basil, finely chopped

3 garlic cloves, minced

½ cup of almonds, roughly chopped

Preparation:

Cook the pasta using package instructions. Remove from the heat and drain well. Set aside.

Place the onions and garlic in a large nonstick frying pan over a medium-high temperature. Stir-fry for 3 minutes and then add broccoli and 1 cup of water. Cook for 10 minutes or until tender. Now, stir in pasta, lemon juice, and basil. Sprinkle some salt and pepper to taste. Add 1 more cup of water and reduce the heat. Cover with a lid and cook until liquid evaporates. Remove from the heat and top with almonds before serving.

Nutrition information per serving: Kcal: 356, Protein: 15.1g, Carbs: 58.9g, Fats: 7.4g

4. Quick Almond Pudding

Ingredients:

3/4 cup of ground almonds

1/4 cup of coconut, grated

3/4 cup of goji berries

1 cup of coconut milk

½ cup of water

1 tsp of vanilla extract

1 tsp of orange zest

1 tbsp of cornstarch

Preparation:

Combine cornstarch, vanilla extract, orange zest, and coconut milk in a deep pot. Cook for about 10-15 minutes on a low temperature. Remove from the heat and let it cool for a while.

Meanwhile, place almonds, grated coconut, goji berries and water in a food processor for 2 minutes. Add cornstarch mixture and grated coconut and mix for another 1-2 minutes.

Pour the mixture into the pudding bowls. Let it stand in the refrigerator for few hours before serving.

Nutrition information per serving: Kcal: 360, Protein: 7.1g, Carbs: 13.3g, Fats: 33.2g

5. Chicken Wings with Turmeric Sauce

Ingredients:

1lb of chicken wings, skinless

1 cup of almond milk

1 tbsp of coconut oil

2 tbsp of almond flour

1 tsp of turmeric, ground

¼ cup of olive oil

½ tsp of dried rosemary, finely chopped

¼ tsp of red pepper, ground

1 tbsp of garlic, ground

Preparation:

Preheat the oven to 300°F.

Combine rosemary, red pepper, garlic and olive oil in a large bowl. Place chicken wings coat in the marinade for about 30 minutes.

Meanwhile, melt coconut oil in a large nonstick saucepan. Add almond flour and stir for few minutes. Remove from the heat and stir in turmeric and almond milk. Return to the heat and cook for about 7-10 minutes over a medium-high temperature.

Remove the chicken wings from the marinade and place on a baking sheet. Bake uncovered for about 20 minutes. Remove from the oven, pour the turmeric sauce over the meat and bake for five more minutes. Serve with vegetables of your choice.

Nutrition information per serving: Kcal: 513, Protein: 34.8g, Carbs: 8.0g, Fats: 38.8g

6. White Beans Salad

Ingredients:

4 cups of white beans, pre-cooked

5 medium-sized onions, diced

2 cups of Romaine lettuce, chopped

2 large tomatoes, diced

2 tbsp of balsamic vinegar

2 tbsp of extra-virgin olive oil

2 medium-sized carrots, chopped

¼ cup of cilantro, chopped

2 tbsp of lemon juice

2 garlic cloves, minced

1 tsp of cumin, ground

1 tsp of sea salt

½ tsp of black pepper, ground

¼ tsp of Cayenne pepper, ground

Preparation:

Combine lemon juice, vinegar, oil, cilantro, cumin, garlic, salt, pepper, and cayenne pepper in a mixing bowl. Stir well and set aside to allow flavors to mingle.

Place the beans in a pot of boiling water. Cook until soften and remove from the heat. Drain well and transfer to a salad bowl. Stir in lettuce, tomatoes, and carrots. Drizzle with marinade and toss well to coat. Refrigerate for 10 minutes before serving.

Nutrition information per serving: Kcal: 332, Protein: 20.1g, Carbs: 57.2g, Fats: 3.7g

7. Veal Steak with Red Pepper Sauce

Ingredients:

1 lb of veal steak, boneless

3 red bell peppers, chopped

3 tbsp of olive oil

4 garlic cloves, chopped

1 small onion, peeled and chopped

1 tsp of dried rosemary, finely chopped

½ cup of water

Cooking spray

Preparation:

Preheat oven to 350°F.

Slightly coat a baking sheet with a cooking spray. Place the meat on a baking sheet and cook for 60 minutes. Remove from the oven.

Preheat the oil in a large nonstick saucepan over a medium-high temperature. Add garlic and onion and stir-fry for 5 minutes until translucent.

Add peppers, rosemary and ½ cup of water (you can add some more water if the sauce is too thick). Bring it to a boil and reduce the heat to minimum. Cook for about 10-15 minutes. Transfer to a serving plate.

Pour the pepper sauce over the meat chops and serve.

Nutrition information per serving: Kcal: 264, Protein: 24.9g, Carbs: 7.7g, Fats: 14.9g

8. Sweet Potato Tagine

Ingredients:

4 small tomatoes, chopped

1 medium-sized onion, sliced

1 medium-sized zucchini, chopped

1 cup of dry apricots

2 tbsp of olive oil

½ tsp of sea salt

2 small carrots, sliced lengthwise

2 garlic cloves, minced

2 tbsp of ginger, minced

1 tsp of cumin, ground

1 tsp of cinnamon, ground

¼ tsp of turmeric, ground

½ cup of water

2 cups of sweet potatoes, peeled and chopped into small pieces

2 tbsp of lemon juice, freshly squeezed

1 cup of canned carrots, pre-cooked and chopped

Preparation:

Preheat the olive oil in a large saucepan over a medium-high temperature. Add the onions and salt. Stir-fry for 5 minutes, or until translucent. Add carrots and fry for another 5 minutes, or until slightly soften.

Now, add the spices and raise the heat. Stir well and add tomatoes, zucchini and apricots. Pour in the water and bring it to a boil. Cover and reduce the heat. Simmer gently for about 20 minutes.

Add sweet potatoes and lemon juice. Cook uncovered until the potatoes are done and the water evaporates. Serve with a cooked carrot.

Nutrition information per serving: Kcal: 138, Protein: 2.5g, Carbs: 23.7g, Fats: 4.6g

9. Orange Carrot Smoothie

Ingredients:

2 large oranges, peeled and chopped

2 medium-sized carrots, sliced

1 cup of Greek yogurt

2 tbsp of honey

1 tbsp of flaxseeds

1 tsp of dried mint, ground

Preparation:

Combine oranges, carrots, yogurt, honey, and flaxseeds in a food processor. Blend until nicely smooth and transfer to a serving glasses. Refrigerate for 30 minutes and top with mint before serving.

Nutrition information per serving: Kcal: 155, Protein: 5.3g, Carbs: 32.0g, Fats: 1.6g

10. Baked Mushrooms in Tomato Sauce

Ingredients:

1 cup of button mushrooms, chopped

1 large tomato, diced

3 tbsp of olive oil

2 garlic, cloves

1 tbsp of fresh basil, finely chopped

½ tsp of salt

¼ tsp of black pepper, ground

Preparation:

Preheat the oven to 300°F.

Wash and peel the tomato. Cut it into small pieces. Chop garlic and mix with tomato and fresh basil.

Preheat the olive oil in a nonstick saucepan over a medium-low temperature. Add tomato and ¼ cup of water. Cook for about 15 minutes stirring constantly, or until the water evaporates. Remove from the heat.

Wash and drain mushrooms. Place them in small baking dish and spread tomato sauce over it. Add salt and pepper to taste.

Bake for about 10-15 minutes, or until doneness. Remove from the oven and serve.

Nutrition information per serving: Kcal: 205, Protein: 2.0g, Carbs: 4.9g, Fats: 21.3g

11. Cheese and Vegetable Frittata

Ingredients:

¼ cup of Cheddar cheese, crumbled

1 cup of leeks, roughly chopped

2 large tomatoes, chopped

1 cup of spinach, chopped

4 large eggs

1 small avocado, sliced

¼ cup of fresh parsley, chopped

vegetable oil spray

½ tsp of salt

¼ tsp of pepper

Preparation:

Spray some oil over a medium saucepan and preheat it to a medium-high temperature. Add leeks and cook about 4-5 minutes, or until soften. Now, add tomatoes and chopped spinach and cook for another 4-5 minutes, until all the liquid evaporates and the vegetables soften.

Meanwhile, whisk the eggs and cheese in a medium bowl. Sprinkle with salt and pour this mixture into the frying pan. Mix well with the vegetables and fry for about 3 minutes, stirring constantly.

Remove from the pan and serve with avocado slices. Sprinkle fresh parsley on top.

Nutrition information per serving: Kcal: 237, Protein: 10.5g, Carbs: 12.1g, Fats: 17.6g

12. Vanilla Rolls

Ingredients:

1 cup of almond flour

2 tbsp of coconut flour

1 tsp of baking soda

2 tsp of vanilla extract

2 tbsp of coconut oil

2 free-range eggs

¼ cup of prunes, finely chopped

¼ cup of almonds, minced

1 tsp of cinnamon, ground

Preparation:

Preheat the oven to 325°F.

Mix together almond flour, coconut flour, baking soda and vanilla extract. Add the eggs and coconut oil. Whisk together until smooth mixture. Set aside.

In another bowl, combine the prunes, minced almonds, and cinnamon. Stir well.

Transfer the dough onto a baking sheet. Roll into a long rectangle and sprinkle with the plum mixture. Cut into 7 equal pieces and let it stand in the refrigerator for about 20 minutes before baking.

Bake the rolls for about 10 minutes, or until nice golden color.

Serve warm.

Nutrition information per serving: Kcal: 160, Protein: 4.3g, Carbs: 19.0g, Fats: 7.5g

13. Buckwheat with Cranberries

Ingredients:

1 cup of fresh cranberries

1 cups of buckwheat groats

1 medium-sized apple, peeled and sliced

1 cup of Greek yogurt

3 egg whites

½ cup of maple syrup

Preparation:

Preheat the oven to 350°F.

Spread the buckwheat groats over a baking sheet and toast for about 5-6 minutes. You want a nice lightly brown color.

Boil the cranberries over a high temperature. Cook until burst. Add the toasted buckwheat groats, egg whites, apple slices, and stir well. Cook for another 7 minutes, or until the buckwheat groats are cooked. Stir in the maple syrup. Remove from the heat and let it stand for 10 minutes.

Top with yogurt and serve.

Nutrition information per serving: Kcal: 375, Protein: 12.7g, Carbs: 78.8g, Fats: 2.3g

14. Green Beans Lamb Chops

Ingredients:

2 lbs of lamb chops

2 lbs of green beans, pre-cooked

2 tbsp of fresh parsley, finely chopped

3 tbsp of olive oil

2 garlic cloves, minced

2 tbsp of rosemary, minced

½ tsp of red pepper, ground

½ tsp of salt

¼ tsp of black pepper, ground

Preparation:

Place the beans in a large nonstick skillet and pour water enough to cover all. Sprinkle with some salt and bring it to a boil. Now, cover with a lid and reduce the heat to low. Cook until soften. Remove from the heat and drain well. Transfer the beans to a large bowl, and stir in 1 tablespoon of olive oil. Toss well and set aside.

Combine parsley, garlic, red pepper, rosemary, and 1 tablespoon of oil in a large glass bowl. Place the meat in it and coat well with the mixture.

Preheat the remaining oil in a large nonstick skillet over a medium-high temperature. Cook for about 5-6 minutes on each side, or until golden brown. Remove from the heat and serve with green beans.

Nutrition information per serving: Kcal: 298, Protein: 34.1g, Carbs: 9.5g, Fats: 13.9g

15. Vegetarian Rice

Ingredients:

1 cup of couscous, uncooked

2 large carrots, sliced

½ tsp of dried rosemary, finely chopped

½ cup green olives, pitted

1 tbsp of lemon juice

1 tbsp of orange juice

1 tbsp of orange zest

4 tbsp of olive oil

½ tsp of salt

Preparation:

Wash and peel carrots. Cut into thin slices. Preheat 2 tablespoons of olive oil in a large nonstick saucepan over a medium-high temperature. Add carrots and cook for about 10-15 minutes,or until soften.Stir constantly.

Add rosemary, olives and orange juice. Mix well. Continue to cook for 3 minutes, stirring occasionally.

Combine lemon juice with 1 cup of water. Add this mixture to a saucepan and mix with remaining olive oil, orange zest and salt. Allow it to a boil and add couscous.

Remove from heat and allow it to stand for about 15 minutes.

Pour these two mixtures into a large bowl and mix well with a tablespoon. Serve.

Nutrition information per serving: Kcal: 443, Protein: 8.4g, Carbs: 53.5g, Fats: 22.6g

16. Spinach Broccoli Quiche

Ingredients:

8 oz of broccoli, chopped

8 oz of spinach, chopped

1 cup of cheddar cheese, crumbled

¼ cup of heavy cream

1 cup of Mozzarella cheese, shredded

6 large eggs

1 tsp of dry mustard

1 tbsp of dill, finely chopped

½ tsp of salt

¼ tsp of black pepper, ground

Preparation:

Preheat the oven to 350°F.

Place spinach and broccoli in a pot of boiling water. Cook for 2 minutes and remove from the heat. Drain well and set aside to cool for a while.

Whisk eggs, mustard, dill, salt and pepper in a mixing bowl. Set aside.

Meanwhile, take a large baking sheet and spread the cheeses on the bottom. Make the next layer with spinach and broccoli. Pour the egg mixture on top. Place it in the oven and bake for about 25-30 minutes, or until set.

Nutrition information per serving: Kcal: 244, Protein: 17.8g, Carbs: 6.4g, Fats: 17.2g

17. Grilled Avocado in Curry Sauce

Ingredients:

1 large avocado, pitted and chopped

¼ cup of water

1 tbsp of curry powder

2 tbsp of olive oil

1 tsp of tomato sauce

1 tsp of fresh parsley, chopped

¼ tsp of red pepper, ground

¼ tsp of sea salt

Preparation:

Preheat the oil in a large saucepan over a medium-high temperature.

In a small bowl, combine curry powder, tomato sauce, chopped parsley, red pepper and sea salt. Add water and cook for about 5 minutes, stirring occasionally. Add chopped avocado, stir well and cook for another 5 minutes, or until all liquid evaporates. Turn off the heat and cover. Let it stand for about 15-20 minutes before serving.

Nutrition information per serving: Kcal: 341, Protein: 2.5g, Carbs: 11.8g, Fats: 34.1g

18. Fried Vegetables with Cottage cheese

Ingredients:

½ cup of cottage cheese

1 small onion, chopped

1 small carrot, sliced

1 small tomato, chopped

2 medium-sized bell peppers, chopped

½ tsp of salt

1 tbsp of olive oil

Preparation:

Wash and pat dry the vegetables using a kitchen paper. Cut into thin slices or strips.

Preheat the olive oil in a large saucepan over a medium-high temperature. Add the vegetables and fry for 10 minutes, stirring constantly. Add salt and mix well. You want to wait until the vegetables soften, then add soft cottage cheese. Stir well. Fry for another 2-3 minutes. Remove from the heat and serve.

Nutrition information per serving: Kcal: 121, Protein: 6.6g, Carbs: 12.4g, Fats: 5.7g

19. Creamy Leeks

Ingredients:

2 cups of leeks, trimmed

1 cup of cream cheese

½ cup of cottage cheese

1 tbsp of olive oil

½ tsp of salt

¼ tsp of black pepper, ground

A few thyme leaves

Preparation:

Cut the leeks into small pieces and wash it under cold water, a day before serving. Leave it overnight in a plastic bag.

Preheat the oil in a large nonstick skillet over a medium-high temperature. Add cottage cheese and cream cheese and fry for about 10 minutes. Add leeks, mix well and reduce the temperature to low. Fry for 10 minutes, or until soften. Remove from the saucepan and allow it to cool. Decorate with thyme leaves. Add salt and pepper to taste.

Nutrition information per serving: Kcal: 380, Protein: 11.9g, Carbs: 12.0g, Fats: 32.5g

20. Tuna with Grilled Eggplants

Ingredients:

1 lb of tuna filets, skinless and boneless

1 large eggplant, cut into bite-sized pieces

2 tbsp of balsamic vinegar

1 tbsp of lemon juice

2 tbsp of olive oil

½ tsp of salt

¼ tsp of black pepper, ground

2 tbsp of tomato sauce

1 tbsp of fresh rosemary, finely chopped

Preparation:

Preheat the grill to a medium-high temperature.

Place vinegar, tomato sauce, lemon juice, 1tablespoon of oil, salt, and pepper in a medium glass bowl. Add eggplant and coat well with marinade. Refrigerate for 10 minutes.

Preheat the remaining oil in a large nonstick skillet over a medium-high temperature. Add meat and cook for 7-10 minutes, stirring occasionally. Remove from the heat, add eggplant chops. Brush the eggplant with remaining marinade constantly. Cook until soften and serve with meat.

Add some extra salt and pepper to taste if needed.

Nutrition information per serving: Kcal: 307, Protein: 31.4g, Carbs: 7.9g, Fats: 16.5g

21. Jamaican Stew

Ingredients:

4 cups of black beans, pre-cooked

1 lb of tomatoes, diced

4 garlic cloves, minced

1 medium-sized bell pepper, chopped

1 large onion, sliced

1 tsp of curry powder

1 tsp of vegetable seasoning mix

1 tsp of thyme

1 tsp of salt

1/4 tsp of black pepper, ground

1 jalapeno pepper, minced

Preparation:

Place the beans in a pot of boiling water. Cook until soften. Remove from the heat and let it stand in water for 15 minutes.

Meanwhile, preheat the oil in a large pot over a medium-high temperature. Add onions and garlic and 2 tablespoons of water. Saute for few minutes until translucent. Now, stir in jalapeno pepper,bell pepper, thyme, curry, vegetable seasoning mix, salt, and pepper. Cook for 5 minutes, stirring occasionally.

Drain well beans and add to the pot. Pour the tomato sauce over and stir to combine. Reduce the heat to low and cover with a lid. Cook for 40 minutes and remove from the heat. Serve.

Nutrition information per serving: Kcal: 189, Protein: 22.0g, Carbs: 66.5g, Fats: 1.6g

22. Zucchini Cream Soup

Ingredients:

4 medium-sized zucchinis, chopped

3 cups of vegetable broth, unsalted

1 cup of skim milk

1 medium-sized onion, chopped

1 large bell pepper, chopped

1 tsp of dried thyme, minced

1 tbsp of vegetable oil

1 tsp of nutmeg

½ tsp of salt

¼ tsp of black pepper, ground

1 tsp of lemon zest

Preparation:

Preheat the oil in a large nonstick saucepan over a medium-high temperature. Add onions and stir-fry for 5-6 minutes, or until translucent. Add bell pepper, thyme, nutmeg, zucchini, salt, and pepper. Cook for 2 minutes more then add vegetable broth. Cook for the next 15 minutes, or until vegetables tender.

Remove from the heat and let it cool for a while. Transfer to a food processor and blend until smooth mixture.

Return to the pot and add milk. Reduce the heat to low and cover with a lid. Cook for about 15-20 minutes, or until set.

Serve.

Nutrition information per serving: Kcal: 69, Protein: 4.4g, Carbs: 7.8g, Fats: 2.6g

23. Shrimp Pasta

Ingredients:

1 lb of pasta, pre-cooked

2 lb of shrimps, peeled and deveined

2 large bell peppers, chopped

5 garlic cloves, minced

4 tbsp of olive oil

¼ cup of fresh parsley, finely chopped

5 tbsp of lemon juice

1 tsp of salt

½ tsp of black pepper, ground

Preparation:

Cook the pasta using package instructions. Remove from the heat and drain well.

Preheat the oil in a large nonstick skillet over a medium-high temperature. Add shrimps and cook for 2 minutes. Add lemon juice, parsley, bell peppers and stir well. Sprinkle with some salt and pepper to taste. Cook for another 10 minutes, or until set. Remove from the heat and serve with pasta. Sprinkle with oregano and serve immediately.

Nutrition information per serving: Kcal: 374, Protein: 32.8g, Carbs: 36.0g, Fats: 10.4g

24. Asian Turkey

Ingredients:

1 lb of turkey breasts, skinless and boneless

1 tbsp of yellow mustard

1 garlic clove, minced

2 tbsp of maple syrup

1 tbsp of green tea

1 tsp of ginger, ground

1 tbsp of canola oil

½ tsp of salt

¼ tsp of black pepper, ground

Preparation:

Preheat the oven to 350°F.

Preheat the canola oil in a large nonstick saucepan over a medium-high temperature. Add garlic, ginger, maple syrup, and tea and cook for 3 minutes, stirring occasionally. Sprinkle with some salt and pepper to taste. Remove from the heat and transfer the mixture to a large bowl. Add meat and coat well with mixture. Set aside for 20 minutes to allow flavors to penetrate into the meat.

Place the meat with liquid in a large baking dish. Put it in the oven and cook for 30 minutes. Remove from the oven and peel off the skin. Serve with fresh vegetables.

Nutrition information per serving: Kcal: 361, Protein: 39.3g, Carbs: 24.7g, Fats: 11.2g

25. Avocado Lentil Salad

Ingredients:

4 cups of white lentils, pre-cooked, drain, and rinsed

1 avocado, peeled, pitted, and chopped

1 cup of lemon juice

1 medium-sized red onion, diced

2 garlic cloves, finely chopped

1 cup of fresh cilantro, finely chopped

1 tsp of chili pepper, ground

½ tsp of salt

1 tsp of lemon zest

Preparation:

Mix together lemon juice, chili pepper, salt, and lemon zest in a mixing bowl. Stir well to combine and set aside.

Place lentils in a pot of boiling water. Cook until soften and remove from the heat. Rinse with water and transfer to a large salad bowl. Add onion, garlic, and cilantro. Drizzle with marinade and toss well to combine. Top with avocado chops and before serving.

Nutrition information per serving: Kcal: 540, Protein: 34.3g, Carbs: 82.9g, Fats: 8.3g

26. Oven-Baked Shrimps and Vegges

Ingredients:

1 can of tomatoes, diced

1 can of chickpeas, drained

1 lb of shrimps, peeled and deveined

1 medium-sized onion, diced

1 cup of white rice, long-grain

2 garlic cloves, minced

1 small zucchini, chopped

3 cups of chicken stock, unsalted

2 medium-sized bell peppers, chopped

2 tbsp of olive oil

¼ tsp of salt

¼ tsp of black pepper, ground

Preparation:

Preheat the oil in a deep pot over a medium-high temperature. Add onion and garlic and stir-fry for 2-3 minutes or until translucent.

Now, add all remaining ingredients except shrimps. Stir well and bring it to a boil, or until thickened. Remove from the heat and transfer the mixture to a large baking sheet.

Spread the mixture evenly and put it in the oven. Bake for 20 minutes, then top with shrimps. Sprinkle some extra salt and pepper to taste if needed. Bake for another 5 minutes then remove from the oven. Let it cool for a while and serve.

Nutrition information per serving: Kcal: 252, Protein: 18.0g, Carbs: 32.0g, Fats: 5.7g

27. Orange Carrot Soup

Ingredients:

1 lb of carrots, shredded

5 large oranges, chopped

1 cup of chicken broth

3 oz of potatoes, peeled and chopped

2 small onions, chopped

1 garlic clove, minced

¼ cup of Greek yogurt

1 tsp of honey

1 tbsp of olive oil

½ tsp of ginger, minced

5 tbsp of lemon juice

½ tsp of salt

½ tsp of black pepper, ground

Preparation:

Combine lemon juice, mint, salt, and pepper in a mixing bowl. Mix well and set aside.

Preheat the oil in a large nonstick saucepan over a medium-high temperature. Add carrots, garlic, and onions and cook for about 1-2 minutes. Now, add all remaining ingredients except yogurt and bring it to a boil. Reduce the heat to low and cover with a lid. Cook for 15 minutes more and add the lemon mixture. Cook for 5 minutes more and remove from the heat. Stir in yogurt. You can add a few fresh orange chops before serving.

Nutrition information per serving: Kcal: 100, Protein: 2.9g, Carbs: 19.3g, Fats: 1.9g

28. Sunflower Smoothie

Ingredients:

1 large banana, chopped

1 medium-sized pear, cored and chopped

1 cup of Greek yogurt

¼ tsp of cumin

1 tbsp of honey

1 tbsp of sunflower seeds

Preparation:

Combine banana, pear, yogurt, cumin, and honey in a food processor. Blend until nicely smooth and transfer to a serving glasses. Top with sunflower seeds and refrigerate for 30 minutes before serving.

Nutrition information per serving: Kcal: 218, Protein: 11.5g, Carbs: 39.2g, Fats: 3.1g

29. Sweet Potato Oats

Ingredients:

1 cup of rolled oats

1 cup of sweet potatoes, peeled and chopped

¼ cup of dates, pitted and chopped

1 cup of almond milk

1 tsp of ginger, ground

½ tsp of cinnamon

1 tsp of liquid honey

¼ tsp of salt

Preparation:

Place sweet potatoes in a boiling water. Cook until fork-tender and remove from the heat. Drain well and transfer to a food processor. Blend until smooth and place it in a large bowl.

Stir in almond milk, oats, ginger, cinnamon, and honey. Sprinkle with a pinch of salt and mix well to combine.

Transfer the mixture to a medium skillet and cook for 10 minutes. Remove from the heat and stir in the dates.

Nutrition information per serving: Kcal: 597, Protein: 9.9g, Carbs: 75.9g, Fats: 31.6g

30. Cinnamon Strawberry Salad

Ingredients:

½ cup of strawberries, halved

½ cup of blueberries

½ cup of green grapes

1 medium-sized pear, cored and chopped

2 tbsp of lemon juice, freshly squeezed

1 cup of cream cheese

1 tsp of cinnamon, ground

¼ cup of almonds, roughly chopped

1 tbsp of chia seeds

Preparation:

Combine lemon juice, cream cheese, cinnamon, and chia seeds in a mixing bowl. Mix well to combine and set aside.

Combine fruits in a large salad bowl and toss once. Drizzle with dressing and give it a good stir. Top with almonds and refrigerate for 30 minutes before serving.

Nutrition information per serving: Kcal: 284, Protein: 6.2g, Carbs: 14.7g, Fats: 23.5g

31. Mushroom Meatballs

Ingredients:

1 lb of lean beef, minced

2 cups of chicken or beef stock

2 small onions, chopped

2 large eggs

1 cup of skim milk

1 cup of mushrooms

¼ cup of breadcrumbs

1 tbsp of all-purpose flour

1 tsp of vegetable seasoning mix

1 cup of sour cream

½ tsp of salt

¼ tsp of black pepper, ground

Preparation:

Whisk the eggs, breadcrumbs, and milk in a large mixing bowl. Add meat and squeeze with hand to combine.

Preheat a large nonstick skillet over a medium-high temperature. Shape the balls and place into the pan. Cook until browned. Add mushrooms, onions and chicken stock.reduce the heat to low and cover with a lid. Cook for about 25-30 minutes.

Meanwhile, combine flour, sour cream,salt, and pepper in a separate bowl. Stir well and pour the mixture into the skillet. Cook until the mixture thickened. Remove from the heat and serve warm.

Nutrition information per serving: Kcal: 226, Protein: 22.4g, Carbs: 8.0g, Fats: 11.2g

32. Grilled Salmon with Veggies

Ingredients:

2 lbs of salmon filets, skinless and boneless

1 cup of red wine vinegar

2 tbsp of olive oil

2 tbsp of maple syrup

2 garlic cloves, minced

1 cup of green beans, trimmed and chopped

1 cup of cauliflower, chopped

2 small carrots, chopped

½ tsp of salt

¼ tsp of black pepper, ground

Preparation:

Place green beans, cauliflower, and carrots in a pot of boiling water. Cook for 10 minutes, or until soften. Remove from the heat and set aside.

Preheat the oil in a large skillet over a medium-high temperature. Add vinegar, syrup, and garlic. Stir-fry for 1 minute and add meat. Bring it to a boil, then reduce the heat. Cover with a lid and cook for 5 minutes, stirring occasionaly.

Nutrition information per serving: Kcal: 284, Protein: 30.2g, Carbs: 9.1g, Fats: 14.1g

33. Turkey Carrot Salad

Ingredients:

1 lb of turkey breasts, skinless and boneless

5 oz of Romaine lettuce

3 large carrots, grated

¼ cup of Parmesan cheese, grated

5 tbsp of olive oil

1 tsp of Worcestershire sauce

1 tbsp of balsamic vinegar

1 garlic clove, minced

1 tbsp of lemon juice

½ tsp of salt

½ tsp of black pepper, ground

Preparation:

Combine oil, sauce, vinegar, garlic, lemon juice, salt, and pepper in a small bowl or a jar. Mix well to blend. Place the meat into a glass bowl and coat with marinade. Refrigerate for at least 1 hour.

Preheat a large nonstick frying pan over a medium-high temperature. Add meat and cook for 5 minutes on each side. Add carrots and cook for 2 more minutes. Remove from the heat and cut the into bite-sized pieces, or strips.

On a serving plate, make a fine layer of lettuce and top with meat and carrots. Sprinkle with grated cheese and some extra salt and pepper to taste.

Nutrition information per serving: Kcal: 340, Protein: 24.1g, Carbs: 12.4g, Fats: 22.2g

34. Mushroom Wraps

Ingredients:

1 lb of button mushrooms, finely chopped

1 cup of spring onions, finely chopped

1 cup of shallots, finely chopped

1 cup of frozen corn, thawed

2 tbsp of cilantro, chopped

½ tsp of red pepper, ground

2 garlic cloves, minced

1 tsp of ginger, grated

1 tsp of lime zest

½ cup of lime juice

½ cup of cream cheese

1 tsp of mint, finely chopped

½ tsp of salt

4 lettuce leaves

Preparation:

Mix together cream cheese, lime juice, lime zest, red pepper, garlic, and ginger in a medium bowl and set aside.

Preheat a large nonstick saucepan over a medium-high temperature. Add mushrooms, shallots, spring onions and 1 cup of water. Add cream mixture and cook for 5 minutes. Stir in corn, cilantro, and sprinkle with some salt and pepper to taste. Cook for another 2 minutes and then remove from the heat. Let it cool for a while.

Place lettuce leaves on the serving plates and spoon the mixture onto it. Wrap and secure with lid. Serve.

Nutrition information per serving: Kcal: 205, Protein: 8.8g, Carbs: 22.5g, Fats: 11.1g

35. Texas Spicey Spinach

Ingredients:

2 cups of black-eyed peas, pre-cooked

2 cups of fresh spinach, chopped

1 medium-sized tomato, diced

2 cups of corn, kernels removed

2 small onions, chopped

2 red bell pepper, chopped

2 garlic cloves, minced

1 small jalapeno pepper, chopped

For the dressing:

2 tbsp of balsamic vinegar

2 tbsp of olive oil

½ tsp of red pepper, ground

1 tsp of salt

¼ tsp of red pepper, ground

1 tsp of cumin, ground

Preparation:

Mix together all dressing ingredients and set aside to allow flavors to mingle.

Place the beans in a pot of boiling water and cook until soften. Remove from the heat and drain well. Transfer the beans in large bowl. Add remaining ingredients except the spinach and toss well.

Place a handful of spinach on a serving plate. Top with the previously made mixture. Drizzle all with dressing and sprinkle with extra salt if needed. Serve.

Nutrition information per serving: Kcal: 181, Protein: 7.1g, Carbs: 28.5g, Fats: 6.2g

36. Sweet Kale Smoothie

Ingredients:

2 cups of fresh kale, chopped

1 large banana, chopped

1 cup of almond milk

1medium-sized apple, cored and chopped

1 tbsp of honey

1 tbsp of walnuts

Preparation:

Combine all ingredients except walnuts in a food processor. Blend until finely smooth and transfer to a serving glasses. Top with almond and refrigerate for 1 hour before serving.

Nutrition information per serving: Kcal: 322, Protein: 4.5g, Carbs: 35.7g, Fats: 20.9g

37. Creamy Chicken

Ingredients:

12 oz of chicken breasts, skinless and boneless

1 tbsp of butter, melted

½ cup of cheddar cheese, crumbled

½ cup of cream cheese

2 tbsp of fresh parsley, finely chopped

1 tsp of Cayenne pepper, ground

1 tsp of salt

¼ tsp of black pepper, ground

Preparation:

Melt the butter in a large nonstick skillet over a medium-high temperature. Add chicken chops and cook for 10 minutes or until golden brown.

Stir in cream cheese, parsley, and cayenne pepper. Sprinkle with some salt and pepper and cook for 2 minutes. Remove from the heat and let it cool for a while.

Serve with rice, pasta or fresh veggies.

Nutrition information per serving: Kcal: 463, Protein: 40.6g, Carbs: 1.9g, Fats: 32.1g

38. Fennel with Oranges

Ingredients:

2 cups of fennel, trimmed and chopped

5 large oranges, chopped

3 cups of arugula, trimmed

2 cups of white beans, pre-cooked

2 tbsp of lemon juice

2 tbsp of balsamic vinegar

½ tsp of vegetable seasoning mix

¼ tsp of sweet pepper, ground

½ tsp of salt

¼ tsp black pepper, ground

Preparation:

Mix together lemon juice, vinegar, vegetable seasoning mix, sweet pepper, salt, and pepper in a mixing bowl. Set aside to allow flavors to meld.

Place beans in a pot of boiling water. Cook until soften and remove from the heat. Drain well and transfer to a large salad bowl. Add oranges, fennel, and arugula and toss well to combine.

Drizzle the dressing over the salad and serve immediately.

Nutrition information per serving: Kcal: 312, Protein: 17.9g, Carbs: 61.7g, Fats: 0.9g

39. Pumpkin Stew with Cumin Seeds

Ingredients:

1 lb of pumpkin, peeled and chopped

1 medium-sized onion, chopped

2 garlic cloves, minced

2 large carrots, sliced

2 celery stalks, chopped

2 tbsp of tomato paste

1 cup of spring onions, chopped

½ tsp of cumin seeds, toasted

4 cups of vegetable broth

1 tbsp of olive oil

½ tsp of salt

¼ tsp of black pepper, ground

Preparation:

Preheat the oil in a deep pot over a medium-high temperature. Add onions, garlic, and carrot and stir-fry for 3 minutes, or until translucent. Stir in about 2-3 tablespoons of water, cumin seeds, pumpkin chops, and tomato paste. Pour the vegetable broth and stir all well. Reduce the heat to low and cover with a lid. Simmer for 40 minutes, or until pumpkin is fork-tender.

Now, add celery, and cook for 5 minutes more. Remove from the heat and top with spring onions. Serve.

Nutrition information per serving: Kcal: 86, Protein: 3.8g, Carbs: 10.3g, Fats: 2.7g

40. Baked Maple Apple Crisps

Ingredients:

3 lbs of green apples, cored and sliced

1 tsp of cinnamon, ground

1 tsp of ginger, ground

2 tbsp of cornstarch

1 tsp of maple syrup

For the topping:

1 tsp of maple syrup

1 tbsp of honey

3 tbsp of butter

½ tsp of cinnamon, ground

2 tbsp of applesauce

1 tsp of vanilla extract

1 cup of rolled oats

½ tsp of salt

Preparation:

Preheat the oven to 375°F.

Combine apples, ginger, cornstarch, maple syrup, honey, and cinnamon in a large bowl. Stir well to coat the apples.

Mix together all topping ingredients in a large bowl. Stir well to combine.

Spread the apple mixture on a large baking sheet. Add another layer of topping mixture and put it in the oven. Bake for 15 minutes then reduce the temperature to 350°F. Bake until golden brown.

Nutrition information per serving: Kcal: 145, Protein: 1.7g, Carbs: 24.6g, Fats: 5.2g

41. Almond Muesli

Ingredients:

1 cup of rolled oats

2 tbsp of almonds, roughly chopped

½ cup of dates, pitted and chopped

½ tsp of cinnamon, ground

1 large banana, sliced

½ cup of almond milk

5 tbsp of coconut, toasted

Preparation:

Combine all ingredients except almonds in a large glass bowl. Toss well to combine and refrigerate for 15 minutes to soak. Top with almonds before serving.

Nutrition information per serving: Kcal: 559, Protein: 10.3g, Carbs: 83.6g, Fats: 24.5g

42. Turkey Swiss Chard Rolls

Ingredients:

2 lbs of turkey filets, minced

12 large Swiss chard leaves

1 medium-sized onion, chopped

3 tbsp of fresh basil, chopped

5 garlic cloves, minced

½ tsp of dried thyme, ground

5 cups of vegetable broth

¼ cup of fresh basil, minced

1 tbsp of olive oil

1 cup of white rice, long-grain, pre-cooked

½ tsp of salt

¼ tsp of black pepper, ground

Preparation:

Preheat the oven to 350°F.

Place swiss chard in a pot of boiling water. Cook for 20 minutes until soften. Rinse with cold water and drain well. Set aside.

Preheat the oil in large frying pan over a medium-high temperature. Add meat and spread over the pan. Cook for

10 minutes, then add 2 cups of water. Cook until water evaporates. Remove from the heat and set aside.

Now, place rice in a deep pot and add 2 cups of water. Cook until water evaporates, or until set. Remove from the heat and set aside.

Combine onions, garlic and 2 tablespoons of water in a large nonstick saucepan over a medium-high temperature. Stir in thyme, basil, broth, and rice. Cook until boils, then add meat and stir well. Cover with a lid and reduce the heat to low. Cook for about 20-25 minutes and remove from the heat. Sprinkle with some salt and pepper.

Spread the Swiss chard leafs on a clean surface and spoon the meat and rice mixture in the middle. Roll and tuck the ends. Place the rolls in a deep baking dish and pour water enough to cover all rolls. Cover and put it in the oven. Bake for 25 minutes, or until tender. remove from the heat and serve warm.

Nutrition information per serving: Kcal: 225, Protein: 26.2g, Carbs: 15.6g, Fats: 5.7g

43. Coco-Strawberry Banana Smoothie

Ingredients:

1 large banana

1 cup of frozen strawberries

1 cup of almond milk

1 tbsp of cocoa powder

1 tbsp of honey

1 tbsp of chia seeds

Preparation:

Combine all ingredients in a food processor and blend until smooth. Transfer the mixture to a serving glasses and refrigerate for 20 minutes before serving.

Nutrition information per serving: Kcal: 272, Protein: 3.1g, Carbs: 27.6g, Fats: 20.1g

ADDITIONAL TITLES FROM THIS AUTHOR

70 Effective Meal Recipes to Prevent and Solve Being Overweight: Burn Fat Fast by Using Proper Dieting and Smart Nutrition

By

Joe Correa CSN

48 Acne Solving Meal Recipes: The Fast and Natural Path to Fixing Your Acne Problems in Less Than 10 Days!

By

Joe Correa CSN

41 Alzheimer's Preventing Meal Recipes: Reduce or Eliminate Your Alzheimer's Condition in 30 Days or Less!

By

Joe Correa CSN

70 Effective Breast Cancer Meal Recipes: Prevent and Fight Breast Cancer with Smart Nutrition and Powerful Foods

By

Joe Correa CSN